Mediterranean Diet Breakfast Cookbook

Tasty Recipes to Quickly Lose Weight, Feel Great, and Revitalize Your Health

Maria Greenwood

Table of Contents

Introduction

The Basics of the Mediterranean Diet

The foods that we eat have been known to contribute greatly to how our health turns out. Feeding on unhealthy foods is known to cause a myriad of health issues, including chronic diseases; therefore, the diet that one adopts should be given a lot of emphasis. The Mediterranean diet is considered as one of the world's healthiest diet. It's an eating approach that puts emphasis on eating whole foods that are full of flavor. It's a diet that is abundant in fruits, whole grains, vegetables, legumes and olive oil. The diet also features lean sources of protein, and the red wine is consumed in moderate amounts.

The Mediterranean diet is also one of the top most popular diets, and it's not the type of diet where the end goal is only to lose weight; it's considered more of a lifestyle. It should be adopted as a daily practice and a way of living that's sustainable. The Mediterranean diet incorporates traditional and healthy living habits of people from the countries that border the Mediterranean Sea, such as Greece, Italy, France, Spain, Morocco and the like.

The diet varies by country and the region it is adopted, so it may have a range of definitions. However, it is a diet with high intake of vegetables, legumes, fruits, nuts, beans, grains, unsaturated fats like olive oil and fish among others. It, however, includes lower intake of dairy foods and meat. There are several benefits that have been associated with the Mediterranean diet, such as good health and a healthier heart.

Various research studies have proven that those who put a lot of emphasis on healthy fats, whole grains and fish not only weigh less but also experience decreased risks of heart-related diseases, dementia and depression.

Eating in this way means that one gets little room for consuming the unhealthy junk and processed foods, which normally lead to being overweight and obese

MEDITERRANEAN

BREAKFAST RECIPES

These recipes represent a good start for persons wishing to start or continue using the Mediterranean Diet. The taste will be quite encouraging and always sumptuous for anyone looking for better and healthier choices.

1. Big Omelet with Tomatoes

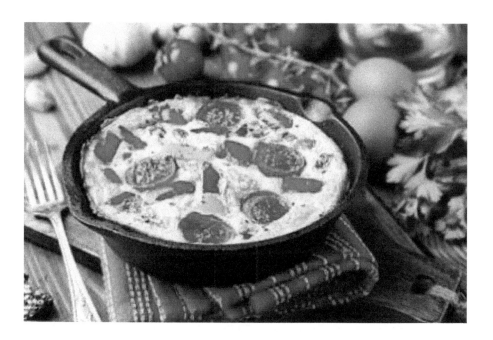

Total Time: 25 minutes

Ingredients:

- 5 eggs
- 3 tomatoes
- 1 bell pepper red or yellow
- 2 oz cheese firm grades
- 3 tbsp milk

- 1 tbsp flour
- 2 tbsp olive oil
- A pinch of salt and spices
- A couple of fresh parsley

Instructions:

1.Wash and dry vegetables. Chop tomatoes into the slices, peel the pepper
and dice it.

2.In a bowl, mix the eggs, milk, flour and grated cheese. Beat by whisk into
uniformity. Season with salt and spices.

3.Heat the frying pan over medium heat. Add oil, fry tomatoes, and pepper.

4.Pour the egg mass into a frying pan, fry under a lid on a slow heat for 15
minutes. Decorate a hot omelet with fresh parsley.

Nutrients per one serving:

Calories: 205 | Fats: 19 g | Carbs: 5 g | Proteins: 17 g

2. Easy Egg Appetizer with Cherry Tomatoes

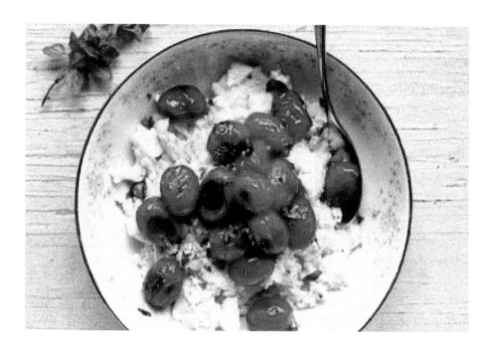

Total Time: 15 minutes

Ingredients:

- 4 eggs
- 10 cherry tomatoes
- 2 tbsp olive oil
- A pinch of dried thyme, spices and salt

- A couple of branches of fresh parsley or cilantro
- 3 oz feta

Instructions:

1.In a bowl, combine eggs, salt, thyme, and spices.
Beat by whisk.

2.Heat the frying pan, add butter, and fry tomatoes for
3 minutes. Lay out into
the plate. Pour eggs into a frying pan and fry in high
heat, stirring by spoon intensively.

3.Lay out egg appetizer on a dish, sprinkle the ground
feta on top, decorate
with tomatoes and chopped greens.

Nutrients per one serving:

Calories: 175 | Fats: 18 g | Carbs: 4.2 g | Proteins: 15
g

3.Scrambled Eggs with Ham

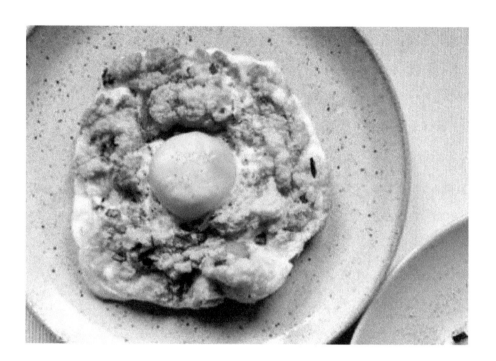

Total Time: 15 minutes

Ingredients:

- 4 eggs
- 2.5 oz ham
- 2.5 oz feta
- 1 green onion
- A pinch of salt

- A pinch of Provence herbs

Instructions:

1.In a bowl, mix the chopped ham, feta cheese, and green onions.

2.Squirrels separated from yolks and beat into a thick foam. Add to stuffing.

3.Cover a baking pan with parchment. Pour protein mass by spoon and make

round cakes with a groove in the center. Add salt and herbs.

4.Bake eggs in a hot oven at a temperature of 220°C 428°F for 4 minutes. In

the center put the yolks and bake for another 2 minutes.

Nutrients per one serving:

Calories: 115 | Fats: 15 g | Carbs: 3.5 g | Proteins: 12 g

4. Oatmeal with Fresh Fruit And Berries

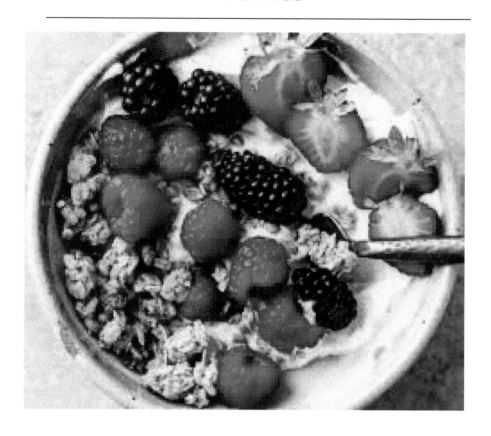

Total Time: 15 minutes

Ingredients:

- 5 tbsp oat flakes
- 1 cup fresh milk

- 1 tbsp honey
- ½ cup fresh fruit and berries to taste strawberry and blueberry

Instructions:

1.Pour milk into a saucepan and bring to boil.

2.Add the oatmeal into the milk, mix and cook for 12 minutes.

3.Pour porridge in a bowl, add honey and fresh fruit. If desired, you can add a

handful of nuts and shavings of dark chocolate.

Nutrients per one serving:

Calories: 124 | Fats: 8 g | Carbs: 3 g | Proteins: 10 g

5.Muesli with Yogurt, Berries, And Fruits

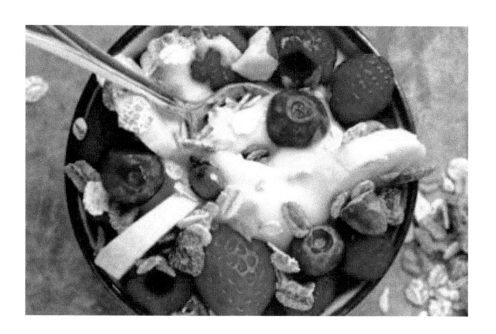

Total Time: 10 minutes

Ingredients:

- ¼ cup muesli
- ½ cup yogurt
- ½ cup berries raspberry, strawberry, and bilberry
- 1 banana

- 1 tsp maple syrup or liquid honey

Instructions:

1.Fill up the muesli into a deep bowl and fill in with yogurt.

2.Lay out the washed berries and pieces of banana; fill in by syrup or honey.

Serve it cooled.

Nutrients per one serving:

Calories: 102 | Fats: 8 g | Carbs: 3.4 g | Proteins: 10 g

6.Cheesecakes with Strawberry

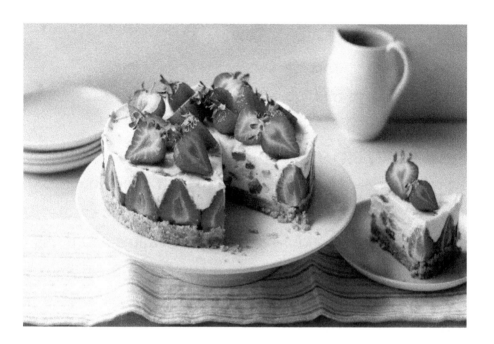

Total Time: 15 minutes

Ingredients:

- 10.5 oz fat cottage cheese
- 2 eggs
- 5 tbsp flour
- 2 tbsp sugar
- 4 tbsp olive oil

- Strawberry for decoration

Instructions:

1.Lay out cottage cheese in a bowl and knead by the fork to uniformity. Add

eggs and sugar, mix well.

2.Add flour and mix ingredients to get the dense dough.

3.Warm a frying pan on a medium heat and pour oil.

4.Strew out a little flour on a flat dish. Divide dough into the necessary amount of cheesecakes and create round balls. Roll in flour ready cheese- cakes and press it by your hand to get flat cakes. Lay out to the frying pan.

5.Fry for 2 minutes from two sides until crust. Lay out on a dish and decorate

with a strawberry. From above you can pour jam or sour cream.

Nutrients per one serving:

Calories: 94 | Fats: 10 g | Carbs: 2.1 g | Proteins: 15 g

7.Cottage Cheese Casserole with Raisins

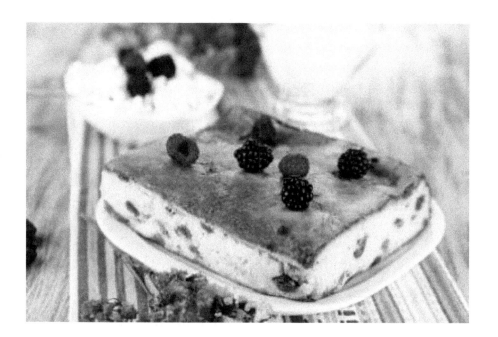

Total Time: 75 minutes

Ingredients:

- 1 tbsp semolina
- 5.5 oz cottage cheese
- 3 tbsp milk
- 3 tbsp sour cream

- 4 tbsp flour
- 1 egg
- 1 tsp sugar
- 2 tbsp raisins

Instructions:

1.Pour the semolina by milk and wet raisins for 7 minutes in cold water.

2.Beat egg with sugar by the mixer to uniformity. Add cottage cheese, semoli-

na, raisins and other **Ingredients**. Mix well. Grease the baking pan.

3.Lay out cheese mass in a baking pan. Grease top of the dish by sour cream.

4.Bake in the oven at 200°C 428°F for 60 minutes.

5.Lay out on a dish and cut into portions. Serve warm.

Nutrients per one serving:

Calories: 268 | Fats: 19 g | Carbs: 4.5 g | Proteins: 18 g

8.Soft Cottage Cheese Mousse with Fresh Berries

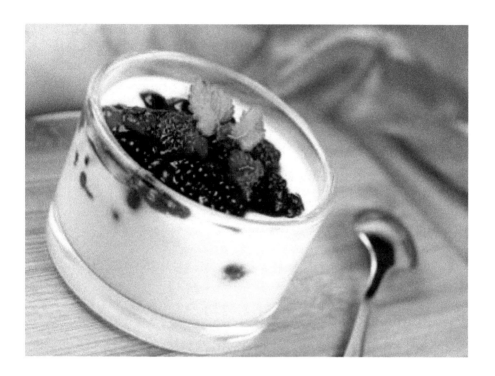

Total Time: 15 minutes

Ingredients:

- oz soft cottage cheese
- 1 cup fresh berries to taste raspberry, blackberry, currant, and blueberry

- 1 tbsp liquid honey

Instructions:

1.Wash berries under cold water. Lay out a half of volume of berries in a stew-

pan and fill in by honey. Simmer for 10 minutes and cool it down.

2.Lay out boiled berries in ice-cream bowls. Beat cottage cheese by a mixer for

receiving dense mousse and layout in ice-cream bowls.

3.Decorate dessert with fresh berries. Serve cooled.

Nutrients per one serving:

Calories: 98 | Fats: 9 g | Carbs: 1.5 g | Proteins: 12 g

9.Berries Smoothie with Muesli

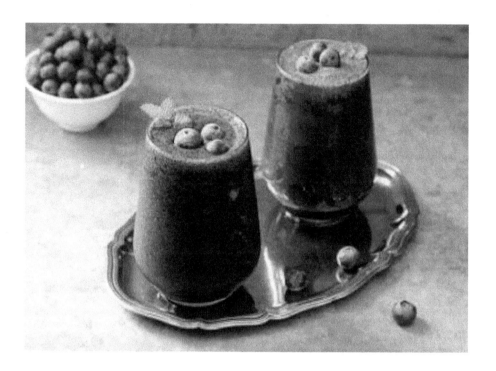

Total Time: 10 minutes

Ingredients:

- 8 big strawberry
- 3.5 bilberry
- 2 tbsp muesli
- 1 cup milk

- 1 tbsp dried fruits raisins, dried apricots

Instructions:

1.Wash strawberry carefully and remove fruit stems. Wash bilberry and drain
them.

2.Put berries in a blender; add dried fruits, muesli, and milk. Beat at a max-
imum speed of 2 minutes to get homogeneous mass.

3.Pour smoothie into glasses and decorate with bilberry.

Nutrients per one serving:

Calories: 64 | Fats: 5 g | Carbs: 2.2 g | Proteins: 14 g

10. Mediterranean Chicken Wrap

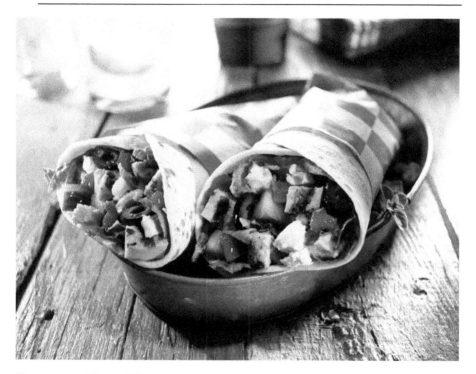

Preparation Time: 5 minutes

Cooking Time: 30 minutes

Ingredients:

- 2 ½ tbsp whole wheat couscous
- ½ pound chicken tenders ¼ cup water
- ¼ cup chopped fresh mint
- ½ cup chopped parsley 2 tbsp lemon juice
- 1 ½ tbsp extra-virgin olive oil

- 1 tsp minced garlic Salt and pepper to taste 2 tbsp chopped tomato
- ½ cup chopped cucumber
- 2 10-inch spinach wraps

Instructions:

1.   In a saucepan, bring water to a boil. Stir in couscous. Remove from heat. Let it stand covered for about 5 minutes. Place aside.

2.   In a small bowl, combine the following **Ingredients**: chopped parsley, chopped mint, lemon juice, olive oil, minced garlic, salt and pepper to taste.

3.   In another bowl, toss the chicken tenders with salt and pepper and 1 tablespoon of the parsley mixture. Place tenders in a non-stick skillet. Cook for 5 minutes in each side over medium heat. Cut into bite-sized pieces when cool.

4.   Combine the remaining parsley mixture with the couscous together with the tomato and cucumber.

5.   Divide and spread chicken and couscous mixture onto each spinach wrap. Roll like burrito. Serve.

Nutrients per one serving

Per serving: 480 calories; 3g saturated fat ,11g monosaturated fat, 64mg cholesterol, 50g carbohydrates, 34g protein, 6g fiber, 652mg sodium; 382mg potassium.

11.   Poached Egg Over Avocado Toast

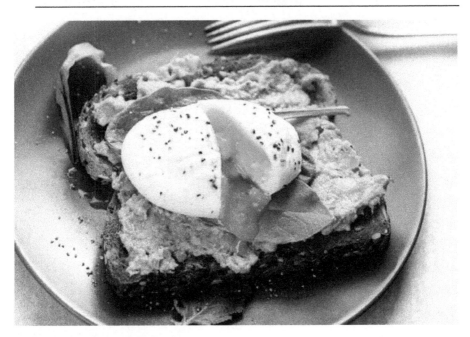

Preparation Time: 20 minutes

Ingredients:

- 1 ripe avocado, halve and stone removed
- 2 eggs, poached
- 2 slices thick whole-grain bread
- 1 tsp lemon juice
- 2 teaspoons olive oil

- Red tomato slices
- Minced chives
- Salt and ground black pepper to taste

Instructions:

1. With your spoon, scoop out avocado flesh into a bowl. Add lemon juice, salt and pepper. Mash roughly with a spoon.
2. Brush bread with olive oil and toast. Spread avocado mixture on each slice. Lay tomato slices and top with the poached egg.
3. Sprinkle with minced chives. Serve.

Nutrients per one serving

Per serving: 445 calories, 31.1g total fat,10.6g sat, 214.1mg cholesterol, 537.7mg sodium, 26.6g total carbohydrates, 7.4g dietary fiber, 2.2g sugar, 16.1g protein.

12. Turkey Potpies

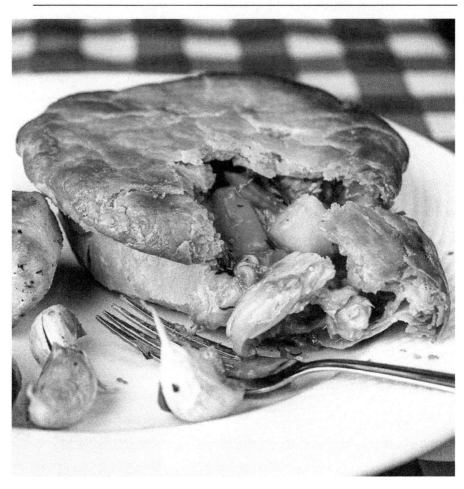

Preparation Time: 30 minutes

Cooking Time: 20 minutes

Ingredients:

- 1 cup cubed cooked turkey breasts

- ½ cup reduced-sodium chicken broth
- 6 oz no-salt-added diced tomatoes, undrained
- 6 oz water-packed artichoke hearts, rinsed, drained, sliced
- 2 tbsp ripe olives, pitted, halve
- 2 tbsp sliced pepperoni
- 2 tablespoons thinly sliced onion
- 1 teaspoon olive oil
- 1 clove garlic, minced
- 1 tablespoon all purpose flour
- Pinch of dried oregano and ground black pepper

crust:

Half a loaf frozen pizza dough, at room temperature or thawed

1 tablespoon egg white

Pinch of dried oregano

Instructions:

1. Using a Dutch oven, sauté onions on olive oil until properly cooked. Add in minced garlic and cook for 2-3 minutes.

2. In a small bowl, whisk together flour and chicken broth until smooth. Gradually stir the mixture to the sautéed onion. Add tomatoes. Bring to a boil and simmer, stirring for 2 minutes until thick. Turn off heat.

3. Add cooked turkey breasts, sliced artichokes, sliced pepperoni, olives, dried oregano and black pepper. Stir gently. Divide mixture among 2 ramekins.

4. Roll out dough to fit each ramekin, cut slits. Place over the filling and press to seal edges.

5. Combine egg white and a pinch of oregano and brush over dough.

6. Place the filled ramekins on a baking sheet and bake at 425 degrees for 20-22 minutes until crust turned golden.

Nutrients per one serving

Per serving: 326 calories, 4g total fat,1g sat, 50mg cholesterol, 699mg sodium, 43g total carbohydrates, 3g dietary fiber, 26g protein.

13. Cheesy Fig-Walnut Crepes

PREPARATION TIME: 20 minutes

COOKING TIME: 5 minutes

Ingredients:

- 3 tbsp plain goat cheese, at room temp.
- 1 ½ tbsp mascarpone cheese, at room temp.
- 1 ½ tbsp chopped walnuts, toasted
- 1 tsp sour cream
- Pinch of salt and ground pepper
- 2 fresh figs, thinly sliced, soaked in Marsala wine for 5 minutes

2 walnut crepes

Instructions:

1. Preheat oven to 350 degrees F.

2. In a small bowl, whisk both cheeses, walnuts, sour cream, salt and pepper until smooth and fluffy.

3. Divide mixture into two. Spread one side of each crepe with the mixture. Arrange slices of fig over the filling. Fold in half or to which shape you prefer. Place in a baking sheet.

4. Bake for 5 minutes just enough to warm them slightly before serving.

Nutrients per one serving

Per serving: 315 calories, 20g total fat,9g sat, 4g mono, 9g poly, 83mg cholesterol, 312mg sodium, 11g total carbohydrates, 2g dietary fiber, 6g protein.

14.   Calli Granola

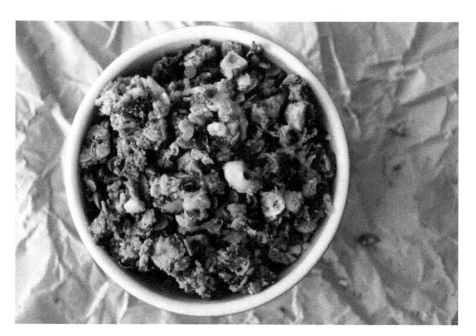

PREPARATION TIME: 10 minutes

COOKING TIME: 30 minutes

Ingredients:

- 1 cup quick cooking rolled oats
- 5 tbsp chopped California walnuts

- ½ cup natural wheat bran
- 2 tbsp honey
- ½ tsp vanilla extract
- ½ cup dried apples
- Fresh fruits for toppings, if desired

Instructions:

1. Preheat your oven to 300 degrees F.

2. In a bowl, stir rolled oats, walnuts and bran.

3. In another bowl, combine honey and vanilla. Microwave on high for 20 seconds until runny. Stir and pour over dry mixture. Toss to coat well.

4. Evenly spread granola in a shallow baking pan. Bake in 300 degree F for 30 minutes until golden. Stir 2-3 times. Cool completely.

5. Stir in dried apples. Top with fresh fruits if desired. Serve and enjoy.

Nutrients per one serving

Per serving: 461 calories, 17g total fat,2.5g sat, 3g mono, 10g poly, 0mg cholesterol, 7mg sodium, 81g total carbohydrates, 13g dietary fiber, 12g protein.

15.   Bell Pepper and Egg Gratin

PREPARATION TIME: 10 minutes

COOKING TIME: 45 minutes

Ingredients:

- Half a whole yellow bell pepper, cut in thin slices Half a whole red bell pepper, thinly sliced 1 small zucchini, thinly sliced
- ½ cup walnuts
- 2 tomatoes, chopped
- 4 thin asparagus spears, cut into 2-inch lengths
- 1 tbsp olive oil
- 2 tbsp sliced onions
- Pinch of red chili flakes, kosher salt and freshly ground black pepper ¼ cup packed basil leaves
- 2 eggs

Instructions:

1. Preheat your oven to 350 degrees F. Place 2 shallow baking dishes on a baking sheet and set aside.

2. In a skillet, sauté olive oil, onions and chili flakes over medium heat. Cook stirring for 3 minutes. Add peppers, continue cooking for 7 minutes. Add zucchini and tomatoes. Cook stirring for 10 minutes until tender. Stir in basil leaves.

3. In a shallow pan, bring salted water to a boil. Add asparagus and cook until firm tender.
Drain and add to the pepper mixture.

4. Divide the mixture into 2 shallow dishes making a well in the center. Break egg and drop into each center.

5. Arrange asparagus around edges. Sprinkle with walnuts. Bake for another 20 minutes, then serve and enjoy.

Nutrients per one serving

Per serving: 400 calories, 32g total fat,5g sat, 10g mono, 15g poly, 0mg cholesterol, 566mg sodium, 21g total carbohydrates, 7g dietary fiber, 15g protein.

16.   Mediterranean Breakfast Plate

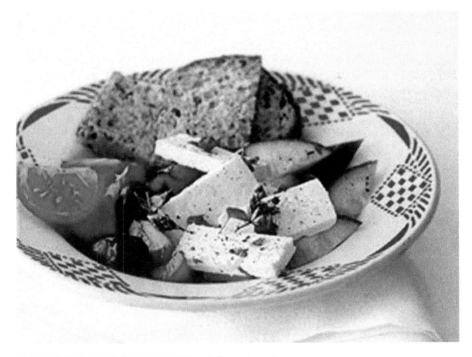

PREPARATION TIME: 10 minutes

COOKING TIME:

Ingredients:

- 2 large tomatoes, cut into wedges
- 4 slices oat, soya, and linseed bread

- 150g cucumber, chunked
- 75g reduced-fat feta cheese, cubed
- 6 black olives
- 4 pcs. onion rings
- 1 ½ tsp olive oil
- Freshly ground black pepper

Instructions:

1. In two serving plate, divide and arrange tomatoes, cheese, cucumber and olives.
2. Sprinkle each plate with olive oil, and pepper.
3. Top with onion rings and bread to serve.

Nutrients per one serving

Per serving: 368 calories, 10g total fat,4g sat 873mg sodium, 45g total carbohydrates, 7g dietary fiber, 10g sugar, 18g protein.

17. Fruity Breakfast Bowl

PREPARATION TIME: 5 minutes

COOKING TIME: 1 minute

Ingredients:

1 cup dried prunes, pitted

1 cup dried apricots, pitted

¼ cup almonds, slivered 2 tbsp water

¼ cup low-fat Greek yogurt

Instructions:

1. In a bowl, mix apricots, prunes and water. Microwave for a minute.
2. Divide evenly into 2 serving bowls and top with yogurt and almonds.
3. Serve.

18. Quinoa Breakfast

PREPARATION TIME: 10 minutes

COOKING TIME: 20 minutes

Ingredients:

1 cup quinoa

2 cups milk

2 dried dates, pitted and chopped finely

2 dried apricots, pitted and chopped finely

¼ cup chopped raw almonds

1 teaspoon each sea salt, ground cinnamon and vanilla extract

2 tbsp honey

Instructions:

1. In a skillet, toast almonds for 5 minutes until just golden brown. Set aside.

2. In another saucepan, heat cinnamon and quinoa together over medium heat until warmed through. Stir in milk and salt and bring to a boil. Reduce heat to low. Simmer covered for 15 minutes and stir in vanilla, honey, apricots, dates, and half of the almonds. Turn off heat.

3. Divide the mixture into two serving bowls. Top with the rest of almonds to serve.

19. Mini Spinach Frittatas

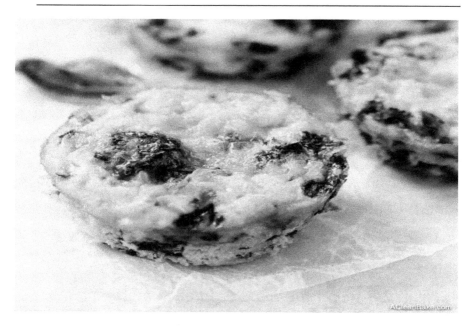

PREPARATION TIME: 15 minutes

COOKING TIME: 30 minutes

Ingredients:

- 3 eggs
- 3 tbsp milk
- 1 tsp chopped onion
- 2 slices turkey bacon, chopped
- 3 tbsp feta cheese

- ½ cup spinach, chopped Salt and pepper to taste

Instructions:

1. Preheat oven to 350 degrees Fahrenheit. With a non-stick olive oil cooking spray, spray a muffin tin.
2. Heat skillet over medium heat. Add onion and bacon and cook until browned. Add spinach and cook until just wilted. Remove from heat and set aside to cool.
3. In a small bowl, beat eggs and add milk and feta cheese. Stir in spinach mixture.
4. Fill in 2/3 full of the mixture in each muffin pan. Allow to bake for 30 minutes until centre bounces back when touched or becomes firm. Serve and enjoy.

20. Turkey Pitas

PREPARATION TIME: 10 minutes

COOKING TIME: 20 minutes

Ingredients:

- ½ lb ground turkey 2 pita pockets
- 3 oz low-fat Greek yogurt ¼ cup feta cheese, crumbled 1 egg
- 1/3 cup loosely packed fresh mint leaves, coarsely chopped and divided 2 cups thinly sliced iceberg lettuce
- 1½ tomatoes, sliced

Instructions:

1. Cut off 1/3 piece of each pita and process in a food processor to make about 4 tbsp pita breadcrumbs.

2. In a mixing bowl, combine the following
Ingredients: turkey, pita crumbs, feta cheese, egg, half of the mint, salt and pepper. Shape mixture into 4 small patties.

3. Heat skillet over medium heat. Cook patties for 10 minutes each side or until browned and thoroughly cooked. Switch off heat.

4. In a small bowl, combine yogurt and the remaining mint.

5. Fill each pita with lettuce, tomatoes, 2 patties and yogurt sauce. Serve.

21. Creamy Oatmeal Bowls with Raspberry Seeds and Honey

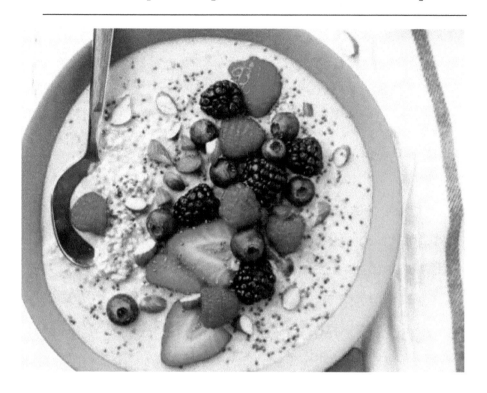

Total Time: 20 min

Ingredients

- Rolled oats – 1 cup
- Ground cinnamon – ½ teaspoon
- Boiling water – 2 cups

- Butter – 2 teaspoons
- Pinch of salt
- For Toppings
- Fresh berries or preferred fruit
- Seeds and nuts of choice
- Honey to taste

Instructions

1. To cook the oats, place a saucepan over medium heat and then add water and sauce and bring to a boil. Add the oats and then cook for about 5 minutes.
2. Lower the heat and allow to simmer for 10 minutes as you stir regularly or until the oats are creamy and water well absorbed.
3. Remove the pot off from heat and then add cinnamon and butter, and cover with a lid as you allow to cook for 5 minutes.
4. Stir the oats again once the 5 minutes are up and then serve topped with nuts, berries and seeds, and drizzle with honey.

Nutrients per one serving

Calories per serving: 541; Carbohydrates: 35g; Protein: 12g; Fat: 26g; Sugar: 0g; Sodium: 450mg; Fiber: 11g

22. Shakshouka Mediterranean Breakfast

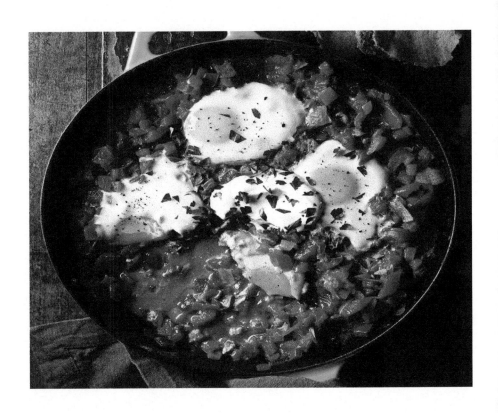

Total Time: 30 min

Ingredients

- Finely sliced onion – 1
- Garlic cloves chopped – 1

- Chopped tomatoes -1 15 oz
- Red bell peppers – 2
- Spicy harissa – 1 teaspoon
- Sugar – 1 teaspoon
- Olive oil – 2 tablespoons
- Chopped parsley – 1 tablespoon
- Eggs – 4
- Salt and pepper to taste

Instructions

1. Place a skillet over medium heat and then add olive oil. After that, add onions and peppers. Cook for about 5 minutes as you stir occasionally.
2. Add garlic and then cook for one more minute. Add tomatoes, harissa and sugar, and cook for 7 minutes. Season with salt and pepper. Next, use a wooden spoon to make about 4 indentations in the mixture and then add an egg to each of the holes.
3. Cover the pot and allow to cook until the egg whites are set. Sprinkle the mixture with fresh parsley.

4. Serve and enjoy with some crusty bread.

Nutrients per one serving

Calories per serving: 455; Carbohydrates: 3g; Protein: 25g; Fat: 38g; Sugar: 0g; Sodium: 350mg; Fiber: 0g

23. Breakfast Casserole with Sausage and Cheese

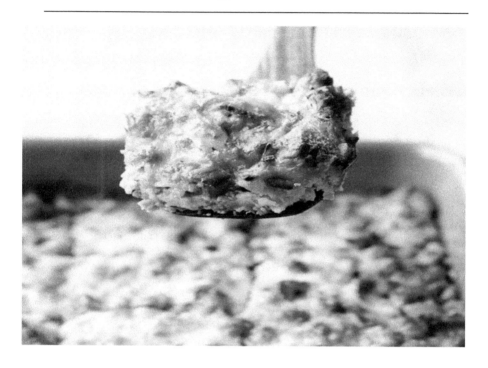

Total Time: 45 min

Ingredients

- Breakfast sausage – 1 pound
- Eggs – 10 large
- Heavy cream

- Cheddar cheese
- Fresh parsley
- Ground dry mustard – 1 teaspoon
- Salt and black pepper ¼ teaspoon

Instructions

1. Have the oven preheated to 3700F.
2. Place a greased skillet over medium heat and then cook minced garlic for a minute or until fragrant.
3. Add sausage and then allow to cook for about 10 minutes or until no longer pink.
4. In a bowl, whisk together the eggs, half of cheddar cheese, parsley, heavy cream, sea salt and black pepper.
5. Have the casserole dish and then arrange the crumbled sausage at the bottom of the dish.
6. Pour the egg mixture over the cooked sausages and then sprinkle with the remaining cheddar cheese.
7. Place in the oven and then bake for 30 minutes or until the cheese is melted and eggs set.

Nutrients per one serving

Calories per serving: 281; Carbohydrates: 1g; Protein: 17g; Fat: 23g; Sugar: 0g.

24. Pancakes

Total Time: 20 min

Ingredients

- Eggs – 2
- Vanilla protein powder – 2 scoops
- Baking Powder – 2 teaspoon
- Liquid stevia – 5 drops
- Pastured butter
- Heavy cream

Instructions

1.   Place all the **Ingredients** apart from butter into a blender. Blend until smooth and well mixed.

2.   Place frying pan over medium heat and then grease with butter.

3.   Add the blended mixture into the frying pan and then allow to cook as you flip once the bubbles appear over the pancake.

4.   Turn the other side and cook as well.

5.   Remove from heat once cooked and then serve in a plate.

6.   Top it up with butter or ghee and then enjoy!

Nutrients per one serving

Calories per serving: 400; Carbohydrates: 1g; Protein: 28g; Fat: 37g; Sugar: 1g; Sodium: 340mg; Fiber: 0g

25.   Mediterranean Toast

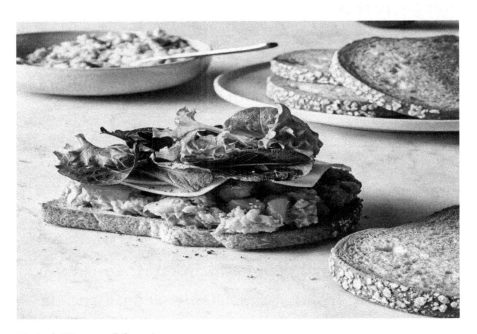

Total Time: 20 min

Ingredients

- Whole-wheat or multigrain bread – 1 slice
- Roasted red pepper hummus – 1 tablespoon
- Mashed avocado – 1/3
- Sliced cherry tomatoes – 3

- Sliced Greek olives – 3
- Hard-boiled egg sliced – 1
- Reduced fat crumbled feta – 1 ½ teaspoon

Instructions

1. Toast the slice of bread and then top with mashed avocado and hummus.
2. Add the cherry tomatoes and olives. Top with the sliced hard-boiled egg and feta.
3. Season with salt and pepper and then enjoy!

Nutrients per one serving

Calories per serving: 333; Carbohydrates: 33g; Protein: 16g; Fat: 17g; Sugar: 3g; Sodium: 730mg; Fiber: 8g

26. Mediterranean Breakfast Egg Muffins

Total Time: 40 min

Ingredients

- Cooking oil spray
- Eggs – 3
- Skimmed milk – 2 tablespoons
- Grated parmesan cheese – 4 tablespoons
- Red pepper finely chopped – ¼
- Chopped tomatoes
- Grated cheddar cheese – 25g
- Leek finely chopped – 35g
- Baby spinach finely chopped – 25g

Instructions

1.   Get the oven preheated to 1900C. Spray silicon muffin tin with the cooking spray.

2.   Whisk eggs, parmesan cheese and milk together in a pouring jug and then season.

3.   Mix all of the finely chopped vegetables into a bowl and then portion into 6 muffin cups.

4.   Pour the egg mixture over each of the muffin cups and then mix with the chopped vegetables.

5.   Divide grated cheddar cheese and use to top each of the muffin cups.

6.   Place in the oven and bake in the center of the oven for about 20 minutes or until the egg is set.

Nutrients per one serving

Calories per serving: 308; Carbohydrates: 9g; Protein: 24g; Fat: 19g; Sugar: 4g; Sodium: 0mg; Fiber: 1g

27.   Mediterranean Omelette

Total Time: 15 min

Ingredients

- Oil or butter – 1 teaspoon
- Milk or cream – 1 tablespoon
- Diced tomato – 2 tablespoons
- Sliced kalamata olives – 2 tablespoons
- Artichoke heart quartered – 1
- Crumbled feta cheese – 1 tablespoon
- Romesco sauce – 1 tablespoon

Instructions

1.   Place a skillet over medium heat. Pour a mixture of milk, egg, oregano salt and pepper and then add to the skillet and cover.

2.   Cook the egg mixture until the eggs begin to set. Sprinkle with artichoke, olive, and feta on the half part

of the egg and then fold the remaining part of the egg over.

3.   Cook the folded egg for about a minute then remove from the heat and top with romesco sauce.

4.   Serve and enjoy!

Nutrients per one serving

Calories per serving: 303; Carbohydrates: 21g; Protein: 18g; Fat: 17g; Sugar: 4g; Sodium: 630mg; Fiber: 5g

28.   Zucchini and Tomato Frittata

Total Time: 15 min

Ingredients

- Eggs – 8
- Crushed red pepper – ¼ teaspoon
- Olive oil – 1 tablespoon
- Thinly sliced zucchini – 1
- Cherry tomatoes – ½ cup halved
- Fresh mozzarella balls – 2 ounces
- Coarsely Chopped walnuts – 1/3 cup

Instructions

1.   Get the skillet preheated. In a medium bowl, whisk the eggs together and then add salt and crushed red pepper.

2.   Heat olive oil in a skillet over medium heat. Add zucchini slices at the bottom of the skillet and cook for about 3 minutes as you turn once.

3.   Top zucchini with cherry tomatoes and then pour egg mixture into the skillet. Top with mozzarella balls and walnuts. Cook for about 5 minutes or until the sides begin to set.

4.   Broil it 4 inches from the heat for about 4 minutes or until set.

5.   Cut into wedges and then serve with slices of tomatoes and basil leaves with additional olive oil.

Nutrients per one serving

Calories per serving: 281; Carbohydrates: 4g; Protein: 18g; Fat: 22g; Sugar: 4g; Sodium: 334mg; Fiber: 1g

29. Blackberry Ginger Overnight Bulgar

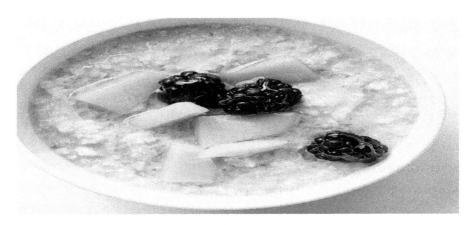

Total Time: 10 min

Ingredients

- Plain low-fat yoghurt – 2/3 cup
- Bulgar – ¼ cup
- Refrigerated coconut milk – 3 tablespoons
- Honey – 2 tablespoons
- Crystallized ginger – ¼ teaspoon
- Blackberries – ¼ cup

Instructions

1.　　In a bowl, stir the **Ingredients** all together apart from the blackberries.
2.　　Divide the mixture into two half jars and then top with blackberries.
3.　　Stir and then serve.

Nutrients per one serving

Calories per serving: 215; Carbohydrates: 4g; Protein: 8g; Fat: 2g; Sugar: 8g; Sodium: 74mg; Fiber: 1g

30. Mediterranean Breakfast Sandwich

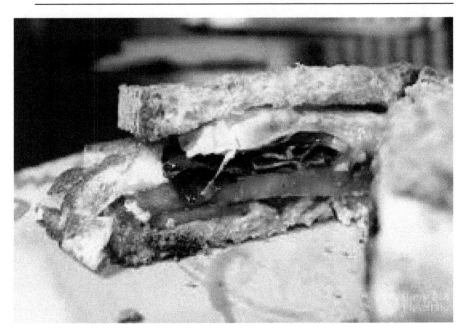

Total Time: 20 min

Ingredients

- Multigrain sandwich thins – 4
- Olive oil – 4 teaspoons
- Fresh rosemary – 1 tablespoon
- Eggs – 4

- Fresh baby spinach leaves – 2 cups
- Medium tomato – cut into thin slices
- Reduced feta cheese – 4 tablespoons
- Kosher salt – 1/8 teaspoon
- Freshly ground black pepper

Instructions

1.   Get the oven preheated to 3750F.

2.   Split the sandwich thins and then brush the cut sides with 2 teaspoons of olive oil. Place the sandwich on a baking sheet and then toast in the oven for about 5 minutes or until the edges are crisp and light brown.

3.   Place a large skillet over medium heat and then add the remaining 2 teaspoons of olive oil. Add rosemary into the skillet and then cook.

4.   Break eggs into the skillet one at a time. Cook for a minute or until the whites are set and the yolks runny.

5.   Break the yolks with spatula and then flip the eggs and cook on one side until well done. After which, remove it from the heat.

6.   Place the bottom halves of toasted sandwich thins onto four serving plates and then top with tomato slices, an egg and a teaspoon of feta cheese.

7.   Sprinkle again with the remaining sandwich thin halves and enjoy.

Nutrients per one serving

Calories per serving: 242; Carbohydrates: 6g; Protein: 8g; Fat: 2g; Sugar: 8g; Sodium: 74mg; Fiber: 1g

31. Eggs with Tomatoes, Olives and Feta

Total Time: 15 min

Ingredients

- Ripe diced tomatoes – 3
- Olive oil – 2 tablespoons
- Pitted and sliced Greek olives – 10
- Eggs – 4
- Grated feta cheese – 1 cup
- Salt and pepper to taste

Instructions

1.   Sauté tomatoes in olive oil for about 10 minutes and then fry in a large pan.

2.   Add olives into the pan and then cook for 5 minutes. In a bowl, whisk the eggs and then add to the

frying pan. Cook the eggs over medium heat or until they begin to set. Add feta cheese and cook to the desired consistency.

3.   Add salt and pepper to taste and then serve and enjoy.

Nutrients per one serving

Calories per serving: 230; Carbohydrates: 4g; Protein: 7g; Fat: 4g; Sugar: 5g; Sodium: 87mg; Fiber: 1g

32. Breakfast Burrito

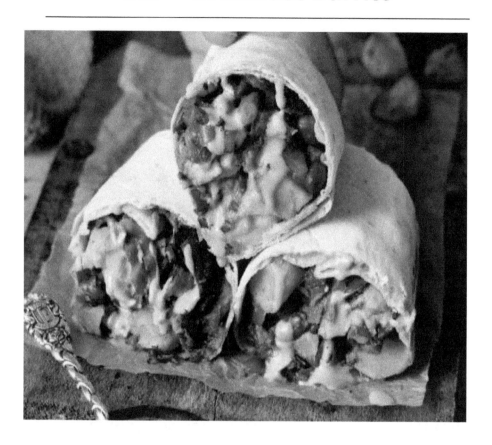

Total Time: 20 min

Ingredients

Tortillas – 6

Eggs – 9

Baby spinach – 2 cups

Black Olives – 3 tablespoons

Sun-dried tomatoes – 3 tablespoons chopped

Feta cheese – ½ cup

Canned refried beans – ¾ cup

Salsa for garnish

Instructions

1.   Use non-stick spray to spray a medium pan and then place over medium heat. Scramble eggs and toss for about 5 minutes.

2.   Add spinach, the sundried tomatoes and black olives. Continue to stir until no longer wet. Add feta cheese and then cover and allow to cook until the cheese is melted.

3.   Add 2 tablespoons of the refried beans on each tortilla and then top with the egg mixture. Divide equally between all the burritos and then wrap.

4.   Grill the burritos in a frying pan until lightly browned and then serve hot with salsa and fruit.

Nutrients per one serving

Calories per serving: 252; Carbohydrates: 21g; Protein: 14g; Fat: 11g; Sugar: 3g; Sodium: 687mg; Fiber: 2g

33. Mediterranean Breakfast Quinoa

Total Time: 25 min

Ingredients

- Ground Cinnamon- 1 teaspoon
- Raw almonds chopped – ¼ cup
- Quinoa – 1 cup
- Vanilla extract – 1 teaspoon
- Honey – 2 tablespoons
- Pitted dates – 2 dried and chopped
- Finely chopped dried apricots – 5

Instructions

1.   Place a skillet over medium heat and then toast the almonds for 5 minutes and set aside.

2.   Place a saucepan over medium heat and then cook quinoa and cinnamon together until warmed through.

3.   Add milk and sea salt to the saucepan and then stir and bring to a boil. Reduce the heat to low and then cover the saucepan and allow to cook for 15 minutes.
4.   Stir in vanilla, dates, honey, apricots and about half of the almonds into the saucepan.
5.   Top quinoa mixtures with remaining almonds and then serve and enjoy.

Nutrients per one serving

Calories per serving: 330; Carbohydrates: 15g; Protein: 14g; Fat: 10g; Sugar: 3g; Sodium:680mg; Fiber: 4g

34. Pancakes with Berries and Whipped Cream

Total Time: 20 min

Ingredients

- Cottage cheese - 200g
- Eggs -   4
- Psyllium husk powder - 1 tbsp
- Coconut oil or butter - 50g
- Toppings
- Fresh raspberries/ blueberries
- Or strawberries - 120g
- Whipping cream - 225mls

Instructions

1.   Put all the **Ingredients** in a bowl and blend to form batter using a wide fork and then leave to expand for 5 minutes to 10 minutes.

2.   Let the butter or oil heat in the frying pan and then fry the pancakes on medium heat for about 4 minutes, flipping carefully. Ensure that the cheese lumps do not stick on to the pan.

3.   Serve with blueberries or the other berries as convenient.

Nutritional Information:

Calories per serving: 80; Carbohydrates: 4g; Protein: 12g; Fat: 36g; Sugar: 1g; Sodium:210mg; Fiber: 0g

35. Mediterranean Frittata

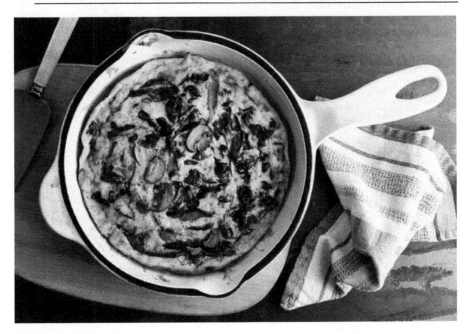

Total Time: 40 min

Ingredients

- Eggs – 12
- Goat cheese – 6 ounces
- Grated parmesan cheese – 1/ cup
- Cremini mushrooms – 4 ounces
- Deli ham – ¼ pound

- Pinch of salt – 1
- Roasted red peppers – 1 jar
- Olive oil

Instructions

1.   Get the oven preheated to 350°F. In a mixing bowl, add eggs, roasted red peppers parmesan, goat cheese and salt. Whisk thoroughly together.
2.   Coat an iron skillet with olive oil and then place over medium heat and add the mushrooms and cook for a minute or until soft.
3.   Add diced ham and then allow it to fry for one more minute. Pour in the egg mixture. Ensure it's well mixed and even.
4.   Transfer carefully to the oven and then let the frittata bake for 30 minutes or until puffy and golden.
5.   Remove from the pan and then allow to stay for a few minutes. After that, cut into wedges and enjoy.

Nutrients per one serving

Calories per serving: 530; Carbohydrates: 5g; Protein: 41g; Fat: 40g; Sugar: 3g; Sodium: 900mg; Fiber: 1g

36.   Breakfast Buns

Total Time: 50 min

Ingredients

- Butter – 3 tablespoons
- Fresh shiitake mushrooms – ½ cup
- Spinach – 2
- Black pepper – 1/8 teaspoon
- Shredded sharp cheddar cheese – 1 ½ cups
- Thin pizza crust – 11 ounces
- Baby spinach – 1 cup
- Fresh sage leaves – 6

Instructions

1.   Get the oven preheated to 400°F and then line the baking dish with parchment paper.
2.   Place a non-stick skillet over medium heat and then add butter, mushrooms and sausage. Cook for

about 4 minutes as you stir frequently until the mushrooms are tender and the sausage thoroughly heated. After that, remove from the skillet.

3.   In a medium bowl, beat eggs and then add salt and pepper. After that, whisk until well beaten. Add butter into the same skillet and then place over medium heat.

4.   Add the egg mixture and then cook for about 3 minutes as you stir frequently until firm and moist. Stir in cheese and then remove from the heat and allow to cool for 10 minutes.

5.   Sprinkle a cutting board with flour. Unroll pizza dough over the board and then press into a 14x10-inch rectangle.

6.   Evenly top with the remaining cheese, eggs and sausage mixture and then press down slightly. Sprinkle the chopped spinach over the eggs evenly.

7.   Begin with the short end and then tightly roll up the dough as you pat the sides to retain the length of about 10 inches.

8.   Pinch the edges to seal. Reshape the buns as you press the tops slowly down. Bake in the oven for about 15 minutes or until golden.

9.   Place a skillet over medium heat and then melt about 1 tablespoon of butter. Add sage leaves and then cook for about 2 minutes as you turn frequently until crisp.

10.   Remove sage to a paper towel and then crumble. Reserve the butter in a skillet. Remove the buns from the oven and then brush the sides with the butter that you have reserved. Bake for a minute longer.
11.   Sprinkle each of the buns with the crumbled sage leaves and then serve them warm.

Nutrients per one serving

Calories per serving: 420; Carbohydrates: 28g; Protein: 21g; Fat: 25g; Sugar: 3g; Sodium:770mg; Fiber: 1g

37.   Celery Egg Sandwich

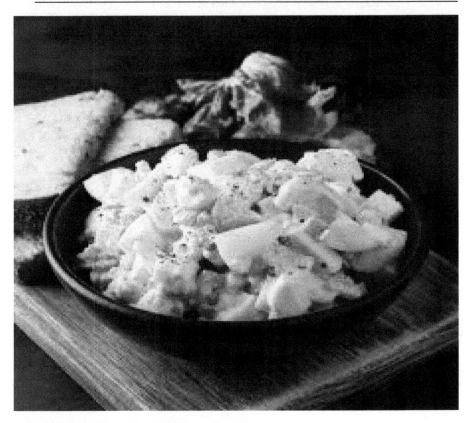

PREPARATION TIME: 15 minutes

Ingredients:

- 2 eggs, hard-boiled
- 2 slices whole grain bread

- 2 tsp olive oil
- ¼ cup plain Greek yogurt 2 tsp Dijon mustard
- 1 stalk celery, diced
- Salt and pepper to taste

Instructions:

1.   Brush each slice of bread with olive oil and toast.
2.   Using a fork, mash the eggs and combine with the remaining **Ingredients** in a bowl.
3.   Place lettuce leaves on top of the bread followed by the egg mixture.
4.   Serve.

Nutrients per one serving

210 Calories, 6g fat, 310mg sodium, 15g carbohydrate, 10g protein.

38. Skillet with Egg, Onion, and Tomato

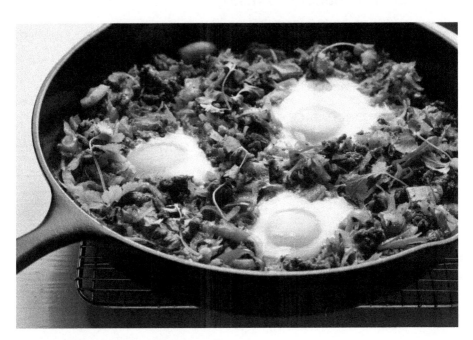

PREPARATION TIME: 28 min

Ingredients

- 1 1/4 c. quartered cherry tomatoes
- 1 tbsp. red wine vinegar
- 2 bunches Swiss chard or rainbow chard

- 2 c. large chopped yellow onion
- 3 tbsp. extra-virgin olive oil
- 4 cloves garlic, minced
- 1/2 tsp. sea salt
- 1/2 tsp. freshly ground black pepper
- 4 large eggs

Instructions:

1. In a small bowl, toss cherry tomatoes with vinegar. Set aside.

2. Remove chard leaves from stems. Chop leaves, place in a large bowl of cool water, and swirl to rinse. Transfer to a colander, allowing a bit of water to remain on leaves. Rinse, dry, and thinly slice stems.

3. In a large cast-iron skillet over medium heat, saute chard stems and onion in olive oil until softened, about 10 minutes. 4. Reduce heat to low. Add garlic and saute 1 minute. Add chard leaves, salt, and pepper. Turn heat to high and toss with tongs until leaves wilt.

5. Using the back of a spoon, make four indents, or "nests," in chard. Crack 1 egg into each nest. Cover the

skillet, reduce heat slightly, and cook until yolks are medium-set, about 4 minutes.

6. Add cherry tomatoes and vinegar to skillet, then serve.

Nutrients per one serving

245 calories, 11 grams, 17 g carbs (5 g fiber), 16 g fat (3 g sat fat), 635 mg sodium

39. Breakfast Sandwiches

PREPARATION TIME: 20 min

Ingredients:
- 4 multigrain sandwich thins
- 4 teaspoons olive oil
- 1 tablespoon snipped fresh rosemary or 1/2 teaspoon dried rosemary, crushed
- 4 eggs
- 2 cups fresh baby spinach leaves
- 1 medium tomato, cut into 8 thin slices
- 4 tablespoons reduced-fat feta cheese
- ⅛ teaspoon kosher salt
- Freshly ground black pepper

Instructions:

1.Preheat oven to 375 degrees F. Split sandwich thins; brush cut sides with 2 teaspoons of the olive oil. Place on baking sheet; toast in oven about 5 minutes or until edges are light brown and crisp.

2.Meanwhile, in a large skillet heat the remaining 2 teaspoons olive oil and the rosemary over medium-high heat. Break eggs, one at a time, into skillet. Cook about 1 minute or until whites are set but yolks are still runny. Break yolks with spatula. Flip eggs; cook on other side until done. Remove from heat.

3.Place the bottom halves of the toasted sandwich thins on four serving plates. Divide spinach among sandwich thins on plates. Top each with two of the tomato slices, an egg and 1 tablespoon of the feta cheese. Sprinkle with the salt and pepper. Top with the remaining sandwich thin halves.

Nutrients per one serving

242 calories; protein 13g; carbohydrates 25g; dietary fiber 6.2g; sugars 3.2g; fat 11.7g; saturated fat 2.9g; cholesterol 214mg;

40. Poached Eggs Caprese

PREPARATION TIME: 10 min

COOKING TIME: 10 MIN

Ingredients:

- Nutrition Facts
- Per Serving: 482 calories; protein 33.3g; carbohydrates 31.7g; fat
- 24.9g; cholesterol 411.6mg; sodium 3092.7mg.
- 1 tablespoon distilled white
- vinegar
- 2 teaspoons salt
- 4 eggs
- 2 English muin, split
- 4 (1 ounce) slices mozzarella
- cheese
- 1 tomato, thickly sliced
- 4 teaspoons pesto
- salt to taste

Instructions:

1.Fill a large saucepan with 2 to 3 inches of water and bring to a boil over high heat. Reduce the heat to medium-low, pour in the vinegar and 2 teaspoons of salt, and keep the water at a gentle simmer.

2.While waiting for the water to simmer, place a slice of mozzarella cheese and a thick slice of tomato onto each English muffin half, and toast in a toaster oven until the cheese softens and the English muffin has toasted, about 5 minutes.

3.Crack an egg into a small bowl. Holding the bowl just above the surface of the water, gently slip the egg into the simmering water. Repeat with the remaining eggs. Poach the eggs until the whites are firm and the yolks have thickened but are not hard, 2 1/2 to 3minutes. Remove the eggs from the water with a slotted spoon, and dab on a kitchen towel to remove excess water.

Nutrients per one serving

482 calories; protein 33.3g; carbohydrates 31.7g; fat24.9g; cholesterol 411.6mg; sodium 3092.7mg.

41. Amazing Blueberry Pie

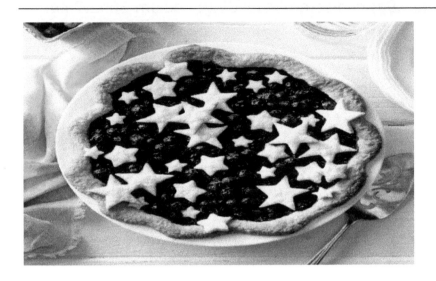

Total Time

Prep: 30 min. Bake: 50 min. + cooling

Makes

8 SERVINGS

Ingredients

- Pastry for double-crust pie (9 inches)
- 4 cups fresh or frozen blueberries

- 1 cup sugar
- 1/4 cup quick-cooking tapioca
- 1 tablespoon lemon juice
- 1/4 teaspoon salt
- 2 tablespoons butter

Instructions:

1. On a lightly floured surface, roll one half of pie dough to a 1/8-in.-thick circle; transfer to a 9-in. pie plate.
2. Trim pastry even with rim; flute edge. Refrigerate 30 minutes. Leave remaining pie dough refrigerated.
3. Preheat oven to 400°. Combine blueberries, sugar, tapioca, lemon juice and salt; toss gently.
4. Let stand for 15 minutes.
5. Add filling to pie pastry; dot with butter. Bake 20 minutes on a lower oven rack.
6. Reduce heat to 350°; bake 10 minutes more.
7. Cover edges loosely with foil to prevent burning. Return to lower rack of oven; bake 15-20 minutes

longer, until blueberries are bubbly and beginning to burst. Cool on a wire rack.

8. Roll remaining dough to a 1/8-in.-thick circle. Cut out stars using different-sized cookie cutters as desired. Place on an ungreased baking sheet. Bake at 350° until golden brown, 5-10 minutes. Remove to wire racks to cool. Place stars over cooled pie in any pattern desired.

42.   Creamy Almond Yogurt

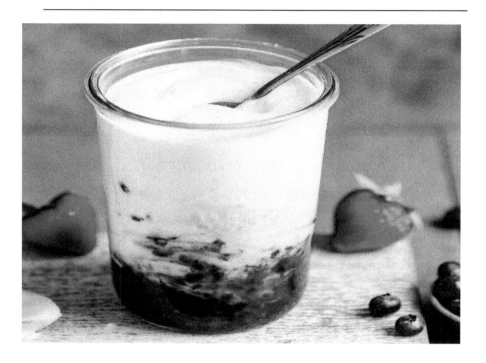

Ingredients

• 1 can Full Fat Coconut Milk

• 2 capsules NOW Probiot-ic-10

• 1/2 tsp. NOW Xanthan Gum (1/4 tsp. split between both jars)

• 2/3 cup Heavy Whipping Cream

• Toppings of Your Choice

Instructions:

1. 1 coconut milk and stir it well. You want to make sure the cream and water in the can is thoroughly mixed.

2. Put the coconut milk into whatever container you'd like. I seperated mine into 2 200mL mason jars. Have your NOW Probiotic-10 handy.

3. Break the capsules into the coconut milk. If you are using 2 jars, use 1 capsule per jar. If you are using 1 jar, use 2 capsules. Stir the mixture togeth-er well and place the lids on the jar.

4. Turn your oven light on and place the jars in the oven. Close the oven door, keeping the light on, and let it sit for 12-24 hours overnight. The longer the bacteria can culture, the thicker the mixture will get, but it doesn't make too big of a difference.

5. Empty all of your yogurt into a mixing bowl and sprinkle 1/2 tsp. Xanthan gum over it. Using a hand mixer, mix this well.

6. In a separate bowl, whip up 2/3 cup heavy cream until stiff peaks form. You want this to be solid cream almost.

7. Dump the solid cream into the yogurt and mix on a low speed until the consistency you want is achieved.

8. Add toppings, flavorings, or fillings of your choice and enjoy!

Usually yogurt has a serving size of 1/2 cup, but you will get just over 1/2 cup per serving with this.

Nutritional Information

315 Calories, 31.3g Fats, 4.3g Net Carbs and 0g Protein.

43.   Caramel Pecan Pumpkin Cake

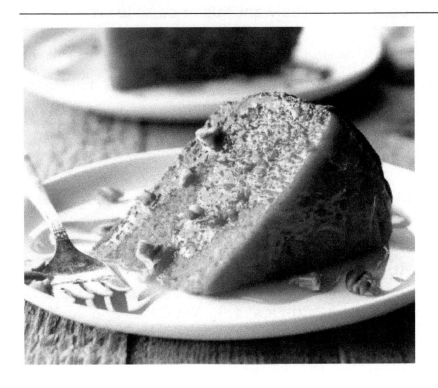

Total Time

Prep: 15 min. Cook: 2 hours

Makes

10 SERVINGS

Ingredients

- 1 cup butter, softened
- 1-1/4 cups sugar
- 4 large eggs, room temperature
- 2 cups all-purpose flour
- 2 teaspoons baking powder
- 1 teaspoon baking soda
- 1 teaspoon pumpkin pie spice or ground cinnamon
- 1/2 teaspoon salt
- 1 can (15 ounces) pumpkin
- 1/2 cup caramel sundae syrup
- 1/2 cup chopped pecans

Instructions:

1. In large bowl, cream butter and sugar until light and fluffy. Add eggs, 1 at a time, beating well after each addition.
2. In another bowl, whisk together the next 5 ingredients; add to creamed mixture alternately with pumpkin, beating well after each addition.

3. Line a 5-qt. round slow cooker with heavy duty foil extending over sides; spray with cooking spray.

4. Spread batter evenly into slow cooker.

5. Cook, covered, on high, until a toothpick inserted in center comes out clean, about 2 hours.

6. To avoid scorching, rotate slow cooker insert one-half turn midway through cooking, lifting carefully with oven mitts.

7. Turn off slow cooker; let stand, uncovered, 10 minutes.

8. Using foil, carefully lift cake out of slow cooker and invert onto a serving plate.

9. Drizzle caramel syrup over cake; top with pecans. Serve warm.

Nutritional Information

1 slice: 473 calories, 25g fat (13g saturated fat), 123mg cholesterol, 561mg sodium, 59g carbohydrate (35g sugars, 2g fiber), 7g protein.

44.   Breadstick Pizza

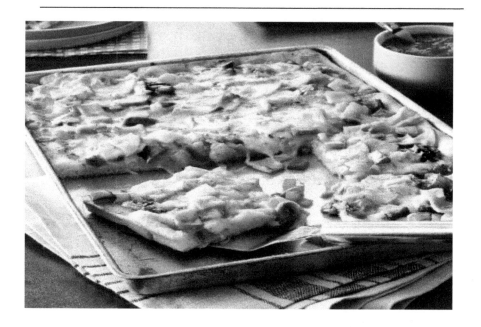

Prep: 25 min. Bake: 20 min. Makes 12 SERVINGS

Ingredients

- 2 tubes (11 ounces each) refrigerated breadsticks
- 1/2 pound sliced fresh mushrooms
- 2 medium green peppers, chopped
- 1 medium onion, chopped
- 1-1/2 teaspoons Italian seasoning, divided
- 4 teaspoons olive oil, divided

- 1-1/2 cups shredded cheddar cheese, divided
- 5 ounces Canadian bacon, chopped
- 1-1/2 cups shredded part-skim mozzarella cheese
- Marinara sauce

Instructions:

1. Unroll breadsticks into a greased 15x10x1-in. baking pan. Press onto the bottom and up the sides of pan; pinch seams to seal.
2. Bake at 350° until set, 6-8 minutes.
3. Meanwhile, in a large skillet, saute the mushrooms, peppers, onion and 1 teaspoon Italian seasoning in 2 teaspoons oil until crisp-tender; drain.
4. Brush crust with remaining oil. Sprinkle with 3/4 cup cheddar cheese; top with vegetable mixture and Canadian bacon.
5. Combine mozzarella cheese and remaining cheddar cheese; sprinkle over top. Sprinkle with remaining Italian seasoning.
6. Bake until cheese is melted and crust is golden brown, 20-25 minutes. Serve with marinara sauce.

7. Freeze option: Bake crust as directed, add toppings and cool. Securely wrap and freeze unbaked pizza.

8. To use, unwrap pizza; bake as directed, increasing time as necessary.

Nutritional Information

1 piece (calculated without marinara sauce): 267 calories, 11g fat (6g saturated fat), 27mg cholesterol, 638mg sodium, 29g carbohydrate (5g sugars, 2g fiber), 13g protein.

45.   Summer Dessert Pizza

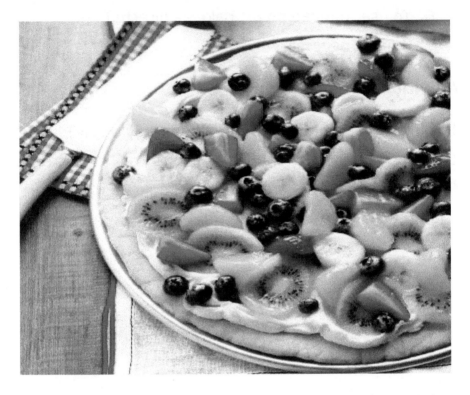

Prep: 35 min. + chilling Bake: 15 min. + cooling Makes 12-16 SERVINGS

Ingredients

- 1/4 cup butter, softened
- 1/2 cup sugar

- 1 large egg
- 1/4 teaspoon vanilla extract
- 1/4 teaspoon lemon extract
- 1-1/4 cups all-purpose flour
- 1/4 teaspoon baking powder
- 1/4 teaspoon baking soda
- 1/4 teaspoon salt
- GLAZE:
- 1/4 cup sugar
- 2 teaspoons cornstarch
- 1/4 cup water
- 1/4 cup orange juice

TOPPING:

- 4 ounces cream cheese, softened
- 1/4 cup confectioners' sugar
- 1 cup whipped topping
- 1 firm banana, sliced
- 1 cup sliced fresh strawberries
- 1 can (8 ounces) mandarin oranges, drained
- 2 kiwifruit, peeled and thinly sliced
- 1/3 cup fresh blueberries

Instructions:

1. In a small bowl, cream butter and sugar until light and fluffy. Beat in egg and extracts.
2. Combine flour, baking powder, baking soda and salt; add to creamed mixture and beat well.
3. Cover and refrigerate for 30 minutes.
4. Press dough into a greased 12- to 14-in. pizza pan. Bake at 350° for 12-14 minutes or until light golden brown.
5. Cool completely on a wire rack.
6. For glaze, combine sugar and cornstarch in a small saucepan. Stir in the water and orange juice until smooth.
7. Bring to a boil; cook and stir for 1-2 minutes or until thickened. Cool to room temperature, about 30 minutes.
8. For topping, in a small bowl, beat cream cheese and confectioners' sugar until smooth.
9. Add whipped topping; mix well. Spread over crust. Arrange fruit on top. Brush glaze over fruit. Store in the refrigerator.

Nutritional information :

1 piece: 176 calories, 7g fat (4g saturated fat), 29mg cholesterol, 118mg sodium, 27g carbohydrate (17g sugars, 1g fiber), 2g protein.

46.   Patriotic Taco Salad

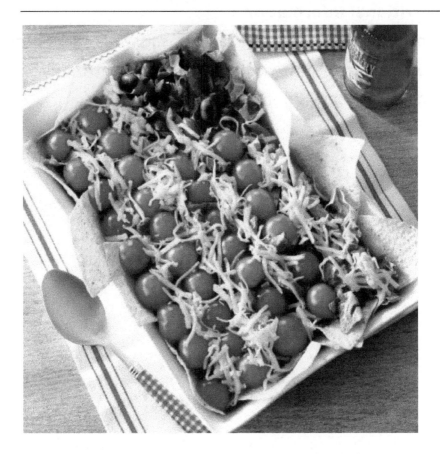

Prep: 10 min. Cook: 20 min. Makes 8 SERVINGS

Ingredients:

- 1 pound ground beef

- 1 medium onion, chopped
- 1-1/2 cups water
- 1 can (6 ounces) tomato paste
- 1 envelope taco seasoning
- 6 cups tortilla or corn chips
- 4 to 5 cups shredded lettuce
- 9 to 10 pitted large olives, sliced lengthwise
- 2 cups Kerrygold shredded cheddar cheese
- 2 cups cherry tomatoes, halved

Instructions:

1. In a large skillet, cook beef and onion over medium heat until meat is no longer pink; drain.
2. Stir in the water, tomato paste and taco seasoning. Bring to a boil.
3. Reduce heat; simmer, uncovered, for 20 minutes.
4. Place chips in an ungreased 13x9-in. dish.
5. Spread beef mixture evenly over the top. Cover with lettuce.
6. For each star, arrange five olive slices together in the upper left corner.

7. To form stripes, add cheese and tomatoes in alternating rows.
8. Serve immediately.

Nutritional Information

1 cup: 357 calories, 20g fat (9g saturated fat), 63mg cholesterol, 747mg sodium, 24g carbohydrate (4g sugars, 2g fiber), 20g protein.

Lightning Source UK Ltd.
Milton Keynes UK
UKHW020722270521
384465UK00005B/102